How to Write an Obituary

A Step-by-Step Guide

HOW TO WRITE AN OBITUARY: A STEP-BY-STEP GUIDE

ISBN 978-0-9813900-3-1

LEGAL DISCLAIMER:

While all attempts have been made to verify information provided in this publication, the authors assume no responsibility for errors, omissions, or contrary interpretation of the subject matter herein.

This publication is not intended for use as a source or legal or accounting advice. The authors want to stress that the information contained herein may be subject to varying state and/or local laws or regulations. All users are advised to retain competent counsel to determine what state and/or local laws or regulations may apply to the user's particular situation.

The purchaser or reader of this publication assumes responsibility for the use of these materials and information. Adherence to all applicable laws and regulations, federal, state, and local is the sole responsibility of the purchaser or reader. The authors accept no responsibility or liability whatsoever on behalf of any purchaser or reader of these materials.

Table of Contents

Introduction

When you've lost a loved one, you are caught up in many powerful emotions. During this time, it can be very difficult to pull together your thoughts to create a lasting tribute in the form of an obituary, but it must be done.

The obituary is much more than a notice that someone has passed away. It is a chance for the family to say goodbye to their loved one, to capture the aspects of that person's life, work, and personality that were most important and that they most want to share with the world.

In this book, we walk you through creating a touching obituary for your loved one, from gathering information, to choosing a format, to writing the actual text of the obituary and submitting it to the newspaper or posting it online, to preserving the clipping of the obituary so it becomes and important part of your family records.

We should tell you now that there are three different kinds of obituary. You may want to create just one, or all three:

A simple *death notice*, which is usually less than 25 words, and includes only the name, age, and location of death of your loved one, and information on the funeral home. Many newspapers will publish a death notice for free if your loved one lived in their distribution area, and it can be a good way to let people know about the memorial service before you have a chance to collect your thoughts and write a full obituary. You can find a template for a simple death notice in the appendix.

An *obituary* may be only a few words longer than the death notice, or it may be up to about 200 words, and may include a photo. Most newspapers charge by the word or by the line, with an extra charge for a photo. In the obituary, you can share details of your loved one's life, and mention the important people they've left behind. You can find templates for several styles of obituary in the appendix. Online memorial sites allow for much longer remembrances, and we've provided links in Sections 5 and 7 for examples of those.

A *memorial* is a notice posted in the newspaper on the anniversary of your loved one's death, one or more years later. It can be a good way for your family to mark an important date, and to acknowledge that though time has passed you are still grieving – and that's okay. You can find templates for memorials in the appendix.

No matter what kind of obituary you plan to create, take your time, and allow yourself to use the creation of the obituary as an opportunity for experiencing and addressing your grief. What you create will be the final tribute to a person who has meant so much to you and many others. And it will become an important keepsake and part of your family records for generations to come.

Section 1

What to Include in an Obituary

Most obituaries are between 50 and 200 words long. How do you summarize a loved one's life in such a short format? It can be a heart-wrenching challenge to decide which parts of your loved one's life are most important to share in their obituary.

Most obituaries include standard information, though of course you can tailor your words to capture the picture of your loved one that is most relevant to you and to others who will read the information.

In Section 5, you'll find examples of obituary formats of different lengths and styles, and we've provided you with templates you can use to create an obituary by simply filling in the appropriate details for your loved one in the appendix. In the coming chapters, you'll find options for poems and bible verses you may wish to include in your loved one's obituary, as well as information on how to contact a charity you'd like memorial donations to go to.

For now, you'll just need to start thinking about the kinds of information about your loved one that are important to you, and that you want to share. This will help you determine which template to use. You may also discover that you need to do some research or gather some records before you continue.

Here are the standard details of a person's life that are usually included in their obituary. If an item is marked as "optional," you can include it in a longer obituary, but it's not required if you prefer to keep things brief.

When you bought this book, you received a Word document called Worksheet.doc, which is a worksheet where you can gather these details easily in one place.

Obituary outline:

- Full name and age: Include maiden name (for example, *nee Jones*) for married women who have changed their name.

- Date and place: Birth date and date of death. You can include the place of birth and death as well, if you choose.

- *Optional* Cause of death**:** You can share this information if you choose, or keep it private.

- Family details: Spouse, children, grandchildren, parents, siblings, or any other family members who were especially important in your loved one's life.

- *Optional* Education: If education was important to your loved one's career, or something that was very meaningful to them, you may wish to include it in their obituary.

- *Optional* Employment/Military service: If your loved one's career was a central part of their life (for example, if they served for 25 years at the same company), or was important to the community (for example, they served on the local city council), you may wish to include it. You can also include information about their military service, if applicable.

- *Optional* Organizations, awards, community contributions, and achievements: If your loved one belonged to any service or community organizations, dedicated themselves to community service, won any awards you'd like to mention, or had any outstanding achievements, you can include them.

- *Optional* Hobbies and interests: If your loved one's hobbies or interests had special meaning in their life (for example, they loved to dance, and this was an important social and emotional center in their life), you can include details.

- Flowers/Donations: Include information on where readers can send flowers or which charity you've chosen to receive memorial donations (more on choosing a charity in Section 4).

- Funeral/Memorial service information: Give the details (date, time, and place) of the memorial service, or simply state that a private service is to be held.

- *Optional* Bible verse or poem: You can include a bible verse or poem in your loved one's obituary to capture your own feelings, or simply to share a verse that they loved (more on choosing a poem in Section 2 and a bible verse in Section 3).

- *Optional* Photo: You can include a photo if you wish. Most newspapers will charge an extra fee to publish a photo, but there may not be an extra charge to publish the photo online. (See Section 6 for how to submit to the newspaper, and Section 7 for how to submit to an online obituary service.)

Section

2

Poems & Quotations to Use in an Obituary

Including a short quotation or part of a poem in your loved one's obituary can be a helpful way to express your feelings. Usually, only a short selection from a poem (a couple of lines) is included in an obituary. You may include a longer section of the poem in a memorial or online tribute.

We have included poems below that are appropriate and touching when used in an obituary or memorial. You may wish to read the poem aloud at your loved one's memorial service as well.

We've also included a number of quotations you may wish to use in your obituary or memorial, or even in your memorial program. You can find appropriate bible verses to use in Section 3.

Poems

She is Gone

You can shed tears that she is gone
or you can smile because she has lived.

You can close your eyes and pray that she'll come back
or you can open your eyes and see all she's left.

Your heart can be empty because you can't see her
or you can be full of the love you shared.

You can turn your back on tomorrow and live yesterday
or you can be happy for tomorrow because of yesterday.

You can remember her and only that she's gone
or you can cherish her memory and let it live on.

You can cry and close your mind, be empty and turn your back
or you can do what she'd want: smile, open your eyes, love and go on.

– *Anonymous*

Until We Meet Again

Each morning when we awake
we know that you are gone.
And no one knows the heartache
As we try to carry on.

Our hearts still ache with sadness
and many tears still flow.
What it meant to lose you,
No one will ever know.

Our thoughts are always with you,
your place no one can fill.
In life we loved you dearly,
In death we love you still.

There will always be a heartache,
and often a silent tear,
But always a precious memory
Of the days when you were here.

If tears could make a staircase,
And heartaches make a lane,
We'd walk the path to heaven
And bring you home again.

We hold you close within our hearts,
And there you will remain,
To walk with us throughout our lives
Until we meet again.

Our family chain is broken now,
And nothing will be the same,

But as God calls us one by one,
The chain will link again

– Anonymous

Remember me when I am gone away

Remember me when I am gone away,
 Gone far away into the silent land;
 When you can no more hold me by the hand,
Nor I half turn to go yet turning stay.
Remember me when no more day by day
 You tell me of our future that you planned:
 Only remember me; you understand
It will be late to counsel then or pray.
Yet if you should forget me for a while
 And afterwards remember, do not grieve:
 For if the darkness and corruption leave
 A vestige of the thoughts that once I had,
Better by far you should forget and smile
 Than that you should remember and be sad.

– *Christina Rossetti (1830 – 1894)*

Life Unbroken

Death is nothing at all
I have only slipped into the next room.
I am I, and you are you:
Whatever we were to each other, we are still.
Call me by my old familiar name;
Speak to me in the easy way you always used
Put no difference into your tone;
Wear no air of solemnity or sorrow;
Laugh as we always laughed
At the little jokes we enjoyed together;
Play, smile, think of me, pray for me.
Let my name be ever
The household word that it always was.
Let it be spoken without effect;
Without the ghost of a shadow on it.
Life means all that it ever meant.
It is the same as it ever was.
There is absolutely unbroken continuity.
What is this death but negligible accident?
Why should I be out of mind because I am out of sight?
I am but waiting for you,
For an interval, somewhere, very near
Just around the corner.
All is well.

– *Henry Scott Holland*

What is Dying?

I am standing on the sea shore.
A ship at my side spreads her
white sails in the morning breeze
and starts for the blue ocean.
She is an object of beauty and I
stand and watch her until at last
she fades on the horizon.

Then someone at my side says
There, she has gone –
Gone where?
Gone from my sight – that is all
She is just as large in the mast,
hull and spars as she was
when she left my side....

The diminished size
and total loss of sight
is in me and not in her,
and just at the moment when
someone by my side says
"She is gone"
others take up the glad shout
"There she comes"

– *Bishop Brent*

Burial Hymn

God of the living, in whose eyes
Unveiled thy whole creation lies,
All souls are thine; we must not say
That those are dead who pass away,
From this our world of flesh set free
We know them living unto thee.

Released from earthly toil and strife,
With thee is hidden still their life
Thine are their thoughts, their works, their powers
All thine, and yet most truly ours
For well we know, where'er they be,
Our dead are living unto thee.

Not spilt like water on the ground,
Not wrapped in dreamless sleep profound,
Not wandering in unknown despair
Beyond thy voice, thine arm, thy care;
Not left to lie like fallen tree;
Not dead, but living unto thee.

Thy word is true, thy will is just
To thee we leave them, Lord, in trust;
And bless thee for the love which gave
Thy Son to fill a human grave,
That none might fear that world to see
Where all are living unto thee.

– John Ellerton

Do Not Stand at my Grave and Weep

Do not stand at my grave and weep;
I am not there, I do not sleep.
I am a thousand winds that blow.
I am the diamond glints on snow.
I am the sunlight on ripened grain.
I am the gentle autumn rain.

When you awaken in the morning's hush
I am the swift uplifting rush
Of quiet birds in circled flight.
I am the soft stars that shine at night.
Do not stand at my grave and cry;
I am not there, I did not die.

– This poem is usually attributed to Mary Frye (1905 – 2004), but has also been attributed to J.T. Wiggins, Marianne Reinhardt, and Stephen Cummins. Some say it is actually a Navajo burial prayer.

Miss Me – But Let Me Go

When I come to the end of my road,
And the sun has set for me,
I want no rites in a gloom filled room,
Why cry for a soul set free?

Miss me a little – but not too long
And not with you head bowed low
Remember the love that we once shared
Miss me – but let me go

For this is a journey that we all must take
And each must go alone.
It's all part of the Master's plan
I'm set on the road to home.

When you are lonely and sick at heart,
Go to the friends we know
And bury your sorrows in doing good deeds,
Miss me – but let me go

– Author Unknown

Crossing the Bar

Sunset and evening star,
   And one clear call for me!
And may there be no moaning of the bar,
   When I put out to sea,

But such a tide as moving seems asleep,
   Too full for sound and foam,
When that which drew from out the boundless deep
   Turns again home.

Twilight and evening bell,
   And after that the dark!
And may there be no sadness of farewell,
   When I embark;

For tho' from out our bourne of Time and Place
   The flood may bear me far,
I hope to see my Pilot face to face
   When I have crossed the bar.

– *Alfred, Lord Tennyson*

Loving Memories

Your gentle face and patient smile
With sadness we recall
You had a kindly word for each
And died beloved by all

The voice is mute and stilled the heart
That loved us well and true,
Ah, bitter was the trial to part
From one so good as you.

You are not forgotten loved one
Nor will you ever be
As long as life and memory last
We will remember thee.

We miss you now, our hearts are sore,
As time goes by we miss you more,
Your loving smile, your gentle face,
No one can fill your vacant place.

– *Author unknown*

God Saw You

God saw you getting tired,
and a cure was not to be.
So He put His arms around you
and whispered "Come to ME."

With tearful eyes we watched you,
and saw you pass away.
Although we love you dearly,
we could not make you stay.

A golden heart stopped beating,
hard working hands at rest.
God broke our hearts to prove to us,
He only takes the best.

– *Author unknown*

For Each Thorn

For each thorn, there's a rosebud...
for each twilight — a dawn...
for each trial — the strength to carry on,
For each stormcloud — a rainbow...
for each shadow — the sun...
for each parting — sweet memories
when sorrow is done.

– *Ralph Waldo Emerson*

The Day God Took You Home

You never said I'm leaving
You never said goodbye
You were gone before I knew it
And only God knew why

A million times I've needed you
A million times I've cried
If love alone could have saved you
You never would have died

In life I loved you dearly
In death I love you still
In my heart you hold a place
No one could ever fill

It broke my heart to lose you
But you didn't go alone
For part of me went with you
The day God took you home.

– Author Unknown

Quotations

"This world is the land of the dying; the next is the land of the living."

– *Tryon Edwards*

"The dark today leads into light tomorrow;
There is no endless joy,
...and yet no endless sorrow."

– *Ella Wheeler Wilcox*

"Death, to a good man, is but passing through a dark entry, out of one little dusky room of his father's house, into another that is fair and large, lightsome and glorious, and divinely entertaining."

– *Macdonald Clarke*

"Look for the rainbow, that gracious thing made up of tears and light."

– *Samuel Taylor Coleridge*

"We think of death as ending; let us rather think of life as beginning, and that more abundantly. We think of losing; let us think of gaining. We think of parting, let us think of meeting. We think of going away; let us think of arriving. And as the voice of death whispers, 'You must go from earth,' let us hear the voice of Christ saying, 'You are but coming to Me!'"

– *Norman Macleod*

"Death is the golden key that opens the palace of eternity."

– *Milton*

"Is death the last sleep? No, it is the last and final awakening."

– *Sir Walter Scott*

Though nothing can bring back the hour
of splendor in the grass, of glory in the flower,
We will grieve not, rather find
Strength in what remains behind.
– *William Wordsworth*

"May the road rise with you, may the wind be always at your back, may the sun shine warm upon your face, and rains fall soft upon your fields, and until we meet again, may God keep you in the hollow of His hand."
– *Traditional Irish blessing*

"When he shall die, take him and cut him out in little stars,
And he will make the face of heaven so fine
That all the world will be in love with night
And pay no worship to the garish sun."
– William Shakespeare, From Romeo and Juliet
(Robert Kennedy read this as part of his eulogy to his brother, JFK)

"We feel so sad when those we love are touched by death's dark hand, but it would ease our sorrow if we could but understand that death is just a gateway that all men must pass through and on the other side of death, in a world that's bright and new, our loved ones wait to welcome us to that land free from all tears where joy becomes eternal and time is not counted by years."
– *Helen Steiner Rice*

"Death and love are the two wings that bear the good man to heaven."
– *Michelangelo*

"When the sun goes below the horizon, he is not set; the heavens glow for a full hour after his departure... And when a great and good man sets, the sky of this world is luminous long after he is out of sight."

– *Henry Ward Beecher*

"What the heart has once owned and had, it shall never lose."

– *Henry Ward Beecher*

"Not by lamentations and mournful chants ought we to celebrate the funeral of a good man, but by hymns, for in ceasing to be numbered with mortals he enters upon the heritage of a diviner life."

– *Plutarch*

"Like some low and mournful swell, we whisper that sad word, 'farewell,'"

– *Park Benjami*

"Every blade in the field,
Every leaf in the forest,
Lays down its life in its season,
As beautifully as it was taken up."

– *Henry David Thoreau*

"Earth has no sorrow that heaven cannot heal."

– *Thomas Moore*

"Death is not extinguishing the light; it is putting out the lamp because dawn has come."

– *Rabindranath Tagore*

"Life is eternal; and love is immortal;
and death is only a horizon; and a horizon
is nothing save the limit of our sight."

– *Rossiter Worthington Raymond*

Section

3

Bible Verses to Quote in an Obituary

The Bible can be an endless source of comfort for those mourning a death and trying to express their feelings in words, even if you are not overtly religious. Here are some of the most searched-for bible verses for use in an obituary or eulogy.

Ecclesiastes 3:1-8

To everything there is a season, a time for every purpose under the sun. A time to be born and a time to die; a time to plant and a time to pluck up that which is planted; a time to kill and a time to heal; a time to break down, and a time to build up; a time to weep and a time to laugh; a time to mourn and a time to dance; A time to cast away stones, and a time to gather stones together; a time to embrace and a time to refrain from embracing; a time to lose and a time to seek; a time to rend and a time to sew; a time to keep silent and a time to speak; a time to love and a time to hate; a time for war and a time for peace.

Ecclesiastes 7:1

A good name is better than a good ointment, and the day of one's death is better than the day of one's birth.

2 Timothy 4:7-8

I have fought the good fight, I have finished the race, I have kept the faith. Now there is in store for me the crown of righteousness, which the Lord, the righteous Judge, will award to me on that day—and not only to me, but also to all who have longed for his appearing.

Matthew 5:4

Blessed are those who mourn; for they shall be comforted.

John 14:2-3

In my Father's house are many mansions: if it were not so, I would have told you. I go to prepare a place for you. And if I go and prepare a place for you, I will come again, and receive you unto Myself; that where I am, there ye may be also.

John 8:12

Jesus said: "I am the light of the world. He that follows me shall not walk in darkness, but shall have the light of life."

John 11:25-26

Jesus said to her, "I am the resurrection and the life. He who believes in me will live, even though he dies; and whoever lives and believes in me will never die.

Matthew 11:28
Come to Me, all you who labor and are heavy laden, and I will give you rest.

Psalm 55:6
Oh that I had wings like a dove! For then would I fly away and be at rest.

Psalm 121:5-8
The Lord watches over you— the Lord is your shade at your right hand; the sun will not harm you by day, nor the moon by night.

The Lord will keep you from all harm— he will watch over your life; the Lord will watch over your coming and going both now and forevermore.

Psalm 23:1-4
The Lord is my shepherd; I shall not want. He maketh me to lie down in green pastures; He leadeth me beside the still waters. He restoreth my soul; He leadeth me in the paths of righteousness for His name's sake. Yea, though I walk through the valley of the shadow of death, I will fear no evil; for Thou art with me; thy rod and thy staff they comfort me.

Revelation 21:4
And God shall wipe away all tears from their eyes; and there shall be no more death, neither sorrow, nor crying, neither

shall there be any more pain: for the former things are passed away.

Philippians 3:20-21
But our citizenship is in heaven. And we eagerly await a Savior from there, the Lord Jesus Christ, who, by the power that enables him to bring everything under his control, will transform our lowly bodies so that they will be like his glorious body.

Romans 8:35-39
Who shall separate us from the love of Christ? Shall tribulation, or distress, or persecution, or famine, or nakedness, or peril, or sword? As it is written "For your sake we are killed all day long; we are accounted as sheep for slaughter"
Yet in all these things we are more than conquerors through Him who loved us. For I am persuaded that neither death nor life, nor angels, nor principalities nor power, nor things present, nor things to come, nor height nor depth, nor any other created thing, shall be able to separate us from the love of God which is in Christ Jesus our Lord.

1 Corinthians 15:54-57
Then, when our dying bodies have been transformed into bodies that will never die, this Scripture will be fulfilled:
"Death is swallowed up in victory.
O death, where is your victory?
O death, where is your sting?"
For sin is the sting that results in death, and the law gives sin its power. But thank God! He gives us victory over sin and death through our Lord Jesus Christ.

2 Corinthians 5:8

Yes, we are fully confident, and we would rather be away from these earthly bodies, for then we will be at home with the Lord.

Revelation 14:13

And I heard a voice from heaven saying, "Write this down: Blessed are those who die in the Lord from now on. Yes, says the Spirit, they are blessed indeed, for they will rest from their hard work; for their good deeds follow them!"

Psalm 116:15

Precious in the sight of the Lord is the death of his saints.

Romans 14:8

If we live, we live to the Lord; and if we die, we die to the Lord. So, whether we live or die, we belong to the Lord.

Section

4

✤ Requesting Donations to a Charity

You may have noticed that many obituaries end with a line that says, "in lieu of flowers, donations may be made to [charity]." When someone passes away, people want to show the family support with some kind of gesture or gift. If your loved one would want your home to be filled with flowers, there is nothing wrong with that. But if you'd like to take the opportunity to request donations be made to a charity your loved one held dear, or that would help you deal with your loss, it's a good idea to mention it in the obituary.

Choosing a charity can be difficult, so it's a good idea to discuss your loved one's wishes with them if you get the chance.

For some, especially those who have passed away after a long or difficult illness, a charity that funds research and care for that illness may be appropriate. For others who have received exceptional care from a particular hospital or hospice, donations may be encouraged to the hospital itself.

Others may wish to support a charity or organization that was important to them during their lifetime, such as the boy scouts, a children's charity, or the ASPCA.

Whatever charity you choose, you should contact them to let them know you are requesting memorial donations be made in your loved one's name. Many charities have web sites with all the information you'll need, but smaller organizations may require a phone call.

Once you've told the charity you're requesting memorial donations, they will be ready to keep an eye out for donations made in your loved one's name. They will compile a list and send you the names of all those who made donations. You may be surprised and comforted to see the names of people you didn't even know had been touched by your loved one. If they were a teacher, you might get donations from former students. Or there might be donations from coworkers you'd never met. These donations often come in with touching notes that the charity will share with you.

Section

5

Obituary Formats & Examples

Once you've gathered all the information you want to include in your loved one's obituary, including their personal information, and poems, quotes, or bible verses you want to include, and information on what charity you'd like to support, you're faced with the difficult task of putting all of that information together into a tasteful memorial notice of your loved one.

You'll need to decide first on a length. Unfortunately, the cost of a long obituary in a major newspaper may be more than you are able to spend. One option is to place a short obituary in the newspaper, and create a longer online memorial web site. You can find information on memorial sites in Section 7.

Then, you need to decide on tone – do you want to be formal, or more contemporary? For some life-long class clowns, a formal obituary just doesn't seem to fit, and it's okay to make the decision to use a tone that respects that individual (though you need to be careful not to go too far).

In this section, we've included nine examples of obituaries in different lengths and styles, each based on one of the templates you'll find at the end of this book.

Example 1: Long, traditional

SMITH, Joanne (nee Jones), 45, of Seattle passed away December 15, 2008 surrounded by loved ones at the Seattle Hospice after a courageous battle with cancer.

Joanne leaves behind her devoted husband John, and their two sons, Jamie and Christopher. She will be sadly missed by her loving sister Sara (Bill) and brother Mike (Jane). Joanne was predeceased by her parents, Gary and Rachel Jones.

Joanne was born in the small border town of Blaine, WA. She was the valedictorian of her high school class, and dedicated her life to the pursuit of education. She received her Master's Degree in Education in 1995 and spent the rest of her life bringing quality education to children in lower-income areas. She received several community awards for her efforts, particularly those focused on making sure inner-city children has access to quality physical education.

Joanne was a dedicated Girl Scouts leader and enjoyed camping, hiking, and exploring nature with the Girl Scouts and her family. In lieu of flowers, donation may be made in Joanne's memory to the Girl Scouts of America.

A memorial service will be held at 1 p.m. on December 22, 2008 at the Home Funeral Chapel.

"You can shed tears that she is gone; or you can smile because she has lived."

Example 2: Mid-length, traditional

This is the same style of obituary as above, with optional details removed to fit a shorter format.

SMITH, Joanne (nee Jones) passed away December 15, 2008 at the Seattle Hospice.

Joanne leaves behind her devoted husband John, and their two sons, Jamie and Christopher. She will be sadly missed by her loving sister Sara (Bill) and brother Mike (Jane). Joanne was predeceased by her parents, Gary and Rachel Jones.

In lieu of flowers, donation may be made in Joanne's memory to the Girl Scouts of America. A memorial service will be held at 1 p.m. on December 22, 2008 at the Home Funeral Chapel.

Example 3: Short, traditional

Again, more details have been removed to shorten this obituary.

SMITH, Joanne (nee Jones), 45, of Seattle passed away December 15, 2008 at the Seattle Hospice. Beloved wife of John. Loving mother of Jamie and Christopher.

Memorial service 1 p.m. December 22, 2008 at the Home Funeral Chapel.

ॐ Example 4: Mid-length, less formal

JONES, Fred. Our beloved father, grandfather, brother, and friend Fred Jones passed away peacefully on September 19, 2008. He was born on June 12, 1927 in Boston.

Fred was predeceased by Sara, his wife of 35 years. He is survived by his three children Roger (Sally), Lou (Margaret), and Ben (Elizabeth). Fred had nine grandchildren, three great-grandchildren, and many other close relatives and friends in Boston and in San Diego, where he spent the last 20 years of his life. He will be greatly missed all.

Fred worked in the Boston school system for 25 years, and later ran a small dry-cleaning business in San Diego. He enjoyed spending time with his family and friends, reading the countless magazines and newspapers he subscribed to, and working in his garden. A memorial service celebrating Fred's life will be held at Home Funeral Chapel on September 26, 2008 at 2:00 pm. For those who wish, the family has requested donations be made to the American Diabetes Association in Fred's memory.

Example 5: Traditional death notice

This is the shortest form of obituary, and many newspapers will publish it for free.

JONES, Fred, 80, of San Diego, September 19, 2008. Memorial service 2 p.m. September 26, 2008 at the Home Funeral Chapel

❧ Example 6: Long contemporary

JOHNSON, Phyllis. 16 September 1925 – 8 December 2008. It is with a deep sense of sadness that the family of Phyllis Johnson announces her quiet passing in Portland, OR, her adopted city since she retired there with her husband in July of 1979. She was predeceased in 1995 by her husband of 40 years, Bob Johnson.

"Ms. P," as she was affectionately known by many throughout the community, will be lovingly remembered by her daughter, Tracy Smith (Paul) of Seattle, WA; and her granddaughter, Susan Peters (Joe) and great-granddaughters Jessica and Natalie of New York, NY. She is also survived by four nieces and nephews and their families, and many, many dear and devoted friends. Phyllis was a woman of deep kindness, and she will be remembered for her constant smile. Fiercely independent, Ms. P played bridge weekly into her final days, and we're sure that she is setting up the bridge table in Heaven.

A celebration of life will be held at 1 p.m. on December 15, 2008 at the Home Funeral Chapel, with a reception to follow. In lieu of flowers, please bring a little sunshine to our world, like Phyllis did, by making a donation to the Humane Society.

"Bury your sorrows in doing good deeds; Miss me – but let me go."

Example 7: Mid-length contemporary

This is the same style of obituary as above, with optional details removed to fit a shorter format.

> JOHNSON, Phyllis. It is with a deep sense of sadness that the family of Phyllis Johnson announces her quiet passing in Portland, OR on December 8, 2008. She was predeceased in 1995 by her husband of 40 years, Bob Johnson.
>
> "Ms. Phyllis," will be lovingly remembered by her daughter, Tracy Smith (Paul) of Seattle, WA; and her granddaughter, Susan Peters (Joe) and great-granddaughters Jessica and Natalie of New York, NY.
>
> A celebration of life will be held at 1 p.m. on December 15, 2008 at the Home Funeral Chapel, with a reception to follow. In lieu of flowers, please bring a little sunshine to our world, like Phyllis did, by making a donation to the Humane Society.

Example 8: Religious Obituary

You can use this example on its own, or add lines from it to one of the other obituary templates.

> JONES, Richard. On August 1, 2008, Richard was called into the arms of the Lord and reunited with his wife Marjorie. He lived a rich live of dedicated service and his testimony will live on. A Memorial Service will be held on August 8, 2008 at the Highland Christian Church.
>
> "God saw you getting tired, and a cure was not to be. So He put His arms around you and whispered 'Come to ME'"

Example 9: Memorial (1 or more years later)

A memorial usually consists of the person's name, their birth and death dates, a quote or verse, and a message of love. Instead of the verse, you can also just write your thoughts.

> James McIntosh. February 12, 1965 – August 12, 2006. We thought of you with love today, but that is nothing new; We thought of you yesterday: and days before that too. We thought of you in silence, we often speak your name: All we have is memories, and your picture in a frame. Your memory is our keepsake, with which we will never part: You are in good keeping; we have you in our hearts. We miss you and love you James, and think of you every day. We will remember you always. Love, your family.

Online Obituary (long):

It is impossible to create a template for an online memorial or obituary, because the format will vary so much based on the life of the individual. In section 7, you'll find links to memorial sites where you can take a look at what other families have created to remember their loved ones.

You may also want to take a look at some of the feature obituaries published in some major newspapers. They are basically profiles and are an appropriate length for an online memorial site. You can find example from the London Telegraph at http://www.telegraph.co.uk/news/obituaries, and from the Globe and Mail (one of Canada's national newspapers) at http://www.theglobeandmail.com/liveslived.

Section 6

How to Submit an Obituary to the Newspaper

One of the toughest questions when it's time to publish an obituary is which newspaper(s) you want it published in. You'll probably want to publish your loved one's obituary in your local community paper, but there may also be a larger metropolitan newspaper, or even a national newspaper.

For example, someone living in the small town of White Rock, British Columbia, Canada, might want their obituary published in the local White Rock paper (The Peace Arch News), the larger metropolitan are newspaper (The Vancouver Sun or The Vancouver Province), and one of Canada's national newspapers (The Globe and Mail or The National Post). You'll need to decide which of these options makes the most sense for reaching the people who would want to know about your loved one's passing.

You may also wish to publish the obituary in the town where your loved one grew up, or an area where they worked for many years or made a major contribution to the community.

Your choice may be made easier by the fact that many newspapers now post the obituary online as a free service when you place an obituary in their paper, which extends the geographical reach of the notice of your loved one's passing. If there are people who you know would want to see the obituary, but who do not live in the circulation area of the newspaper where you've had it published, you can send them information about how to access the online version.

Fees for publishing obituaries vary widely, but are usually based on the length of the obituary and whether or not you wish to include a photo. Some newspapers will publish a free obituary up to a specified length for people who lived in their circulation area. Others will publish a free death notice.

Many newspapers now accept submissions electronically, so check their web site, as this is certainly the easiest way to send it in. There may also be a person at the newspaper you can speak with to get guidelines about pricing and format for the particular paper you've chosen – check the web site or the obituaries section of the paper for a contact number. You may also be able to have your funeral home take care of the actual submission process for you once you provide the funeral director with the written obituary.

If you want to include a photo, the simplest way is to send in an electronic copy, which means you can keep your precious original. If you don't have digital photos, and you don't know anyone who has a scanner, you can take your photo to a business shop like Kinko's and they will scan the photo for you and give you a digital copy on disc. You can either mail the disc to the newspaper, or open it on your computer and send the photo to the paper by email.

You can find detailed information on how to submit an obituary to over 650 American newspapers here: (http://www.legacy.com/Obituaries.asp?Page=SelectNewspapersForHowTo).

All of these newspapers use Legacy.com's online memorial page service, which gives you an online version of the obituary plus an online guest book.

Legacy.com's online memorials stay up for a limited time for free, and you can pay to keep them up for longer. There are a number of paid online memorial sites that will keep your loved one's memorial online for a year, or forever, and offer additional services, such as the ability to light virtual candles in their memory. We'll review five of the top online memorial sites in section 7.

Section

7

Online Obituary Sites & Condolence Books

If you want to share your loved one's obituary with people who live outside of your chosen newspapers' circulation area, you may wish to create an online obituary or memorial page.

As we told you in section 6, some newspapers will include an online version of the obituary and include a guestbook for people to offer condolences, but these online versions offered through newspapers are often only kept online for a limited time – generally 30 days. The advantage of online memorial sites is that they allow you to create a permanent tribute to your loved one, where people's condolences and memories can be a comfort to you forever.

We've reviewed the top five memorial websites online, so you can scan through the information below to choose the memorial site that's best for you. Most memorial sites offer similar features and services, so we've used the following icons to indicate which features each service offers:

- Ability to light virtual candles
- A place for you and loved ones to leave tributes and condolences, or share your memories
- An album where you can upload photos of your loved one
- Ability to add video and/or audio clips
- Ability to create a timeline of events in your loved one's life, or post their biography
- Easy-to-use editing system
- A portion of fees are donated to charity

Parting Wishes

Parting Wishes (www.howtowriteanobituary.com/partingwishes) offers online memorials, as well as will and power-of-attorney tools and forms. Their online memorial service is free for three months, and costs $11 to maintain for a year after that (full pricing options are available on their web site). The site uses an easy wizard that walks you through the process. To access their online memorials, follow the link above, then scroll down to the box that says "Online Memorials."

Christian Memorials

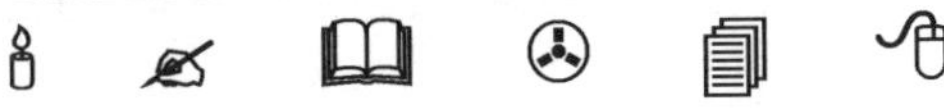

Christian Memorials (www.howtowriteanobituary.com/christianmemorials) offers a free simple obituary page. They offer free 14-day trials on all their packages, which range from basic ($25 – includes basic features and hosting for 12 years) to Premium ($300 – includes all features, 300 mb of storage, and permanent hosting). Sites can be public or password-protected.

Virtual-Memorials.com

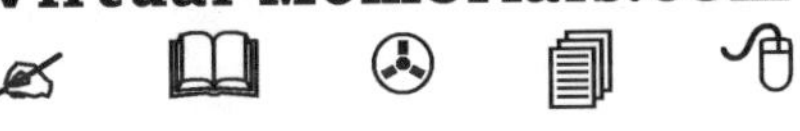

Virtual-Memorials.com has been around since 1996, making it one of the first online memorial web sites. They offer a 14-day free memorial with all of the site's features. After 14 days, the memorial will convert to a basic memorial page, which only includes the text of the main memorial page and any guestbook signatures from the 14-day trial period. If you want to keep the rest of the features, you can sponsor the memorial for $55, or $4.95 per month.

Your Tribute

Your Tribute (memorial.yourtribute.com) has been offering online memorials since 2002. You can create an online memorial with them free for 30 days. After 30 days, it costs $30 to keep your memorial online for one year, or $50 for a lifetime.

Remembered-Forever.org

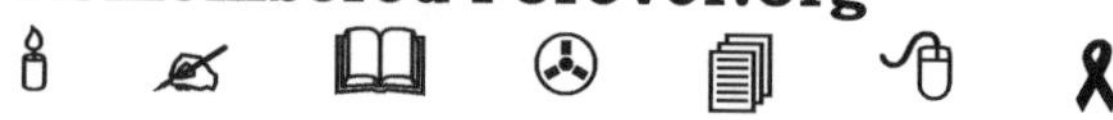

Remembered-Forever.org memorial sites cost $98 for permanent hosting. (They are free for five days.) You can create an online memorial page that is open to the public, or password-protected so that only the people you choose can access it. Even if you don't create an online memorial, you may want to visit their grief support forums at http://www.remembered-forever.org/forum/index.php

iMorial.com

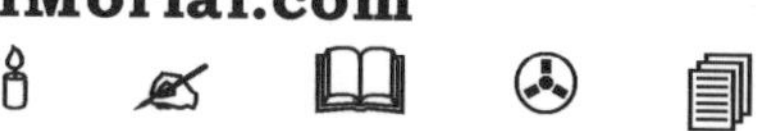

iMorial.com is a free service that offers many of the features of the paid services above. If you're not sure about how well an online memorial will work for your loved one, iMorial.com could be a good place to try it out without making a long-term commitment. If you decide you want to try one of the paid sites, you can always do so later. Memorials on iMorial.com can be public or private.

Memory-Of

Memory-Of (http://www.howtowriteanobituary.com/memory-of) offers a 14-day free hosting period, then has options for monthly ($4.95), annual ($49.95), or everlasting ($94.95) hosting fees. You can also easily create a hard-copy bound memory book from your memorial site.

Section

8

Safekeeping the Obituary

Once you have your loved ones obituary published, you may wish to preserve it for safekeeping. Your loved one's obituary can be a nice summary of their life, and of the things about them that were important and enjoyable to others, so it can be a nice item to pass on to relatives, or keep for a family who has an interest in family records and genealogy.

Newsprint can be challenging to preserve, so it's important to start the process as soon as your receive the newspaper with the obituary published.

First, make a photocopy of the obituary, or scan it into your computer. Regular paper keeps much better than newsprint, so this will be your backup copy.

Next, spray the clipped obituary with de-acidifying spray. You should be able to find this at any craft store that sells scrapbooking supplies. While you're there, you should also buy some acid-free paper, acid-free glue or tape, and a sheet of clear mylar (the clerk at the store can help you identify all of these items).

Once the paper has dried, use the acid-free glue or tape to attach it to the acid-free paper. Then, place the mylar on top. Your loved one's obituary is now preserved as well as it can be, and you can either store it in a file, or place it in an album or scrapbook. If you do place it in an album or scrapbook, be sure to choose one with archival quality, acid-free paper to make sure your loved one's obituary is not damaged.

Final Thoughts

We hope that working your way through this book has helped you to create a meaningful obituary that captures how very important your loved on was in your life. Creating an obituary is an important step in the grieving process, and we hope you have emerged on this side of it feeling confident that you have done your loved one proud.

Appendix

a

Appendix: Obituary Templates

Here are eight templates you can use to help you create a meaningful obituary for your loved one, and one for a memorial. Once you've completed the obituary, please remember to proofread it to check for any typos or other errors. You may also wish to have another family member review what you've written. Then, use Section 6 of the book to submit the obituary to your local newspaper.

Keep in mind that if the exact details of the template don't fit (for example, it mentions a spouse, but your loved one was not married), you can change the details to best fit your loved one.

☙ Template 1: Long, traditional

[LAST NAME], [First name] (nee [maiden name]), [age], of [town] passed away [date] surrounded by loved ones at [location] after a courageous battle with [cause of death].

[Name] leaves behind [his/her] devoted [spouse] [name], and their [children]. [He/she] will be sadly missed by [other relatives (and their spouses)]. [Name] was predeceased by [relatives].

[Name] was born in [town]. [He/she] was [education details]. [Work details]. [Community/Award details].

[Name] enjoyed [hobbies]. In lieu of flowers, donations may be made in [Name]'s memory to [charity of choice].

A memorial service will be held at [time and date] at the [location].

[memorial quote]

☙ Template 2: Mid-length, traditional

This is the same template as above, with optional details removed to fit a shorter format.

[LAST NAME], [First name] (nee [maiden name]), passed away [date] at [location].

[Name] leaves behind [his/her] devoted [spouse] [name], and their [children]. [He/she] will be sadly missed by [other relatives (and their spouses)]. [Name] was predeceased by [relatives].

In lieu of flowers, donations may be made in [Name]'s memory to [charity of choice.] A memorial service will be held at [time and date] at the [location].

Template 3: Short, traditional

Again, more details have been removed to shorten this template.

[LAST NAME], [First name] (nee [maiden name]), [age] passed away [date] at [location]. Beloved [spouse] of [name]. Loving [parent] of [children]. Memorial service [time and date] at the [location].

Template 4: Mid-length, less formal

[LAST NAME], [First name]. Our beloved [relationship], [relationship], [relationship], and friend [name] passed away peacefully on [date]. He was born on [date] in [town].

Fred was predeceased by [spouse/other relatives]. He is survived by [relatives (spouses)]. Fred had [grandchildren/other relatives], and other close relatives and friends in [town]. He will be greatly missed by all.

Fred worked [work details]. He enjoyed [hobbies]. A memorial service celebrating [name]'s life will be held at [location] on [date] at [time]. For those who wish, the family has requested donations be made to [charity] in [name]'s memory.

Template 5: Traditional death notice

This is the shortest form of obituary you can publish, and many newspapers will publish it for free.

[LAST NAME], [First name], [age], of [town], [date]. Memorial service [time] [date] at the [location].

Template 6: Long contemporary

[LAST NAME], [First name]. [Date of birth] – [Date of death]. It is with a deep sense of sadness that the family of [name] announces [his/her] passing in [town]. [She/he] was predeceased in [year] by her [spouse/other important relatives].

[Nickname], as [he/she] was affectionately known by many throughout the community, will be lovingly remembered by [children (spouses)]; and [grandchildren/great-grandchildren (spouses)]. She is also survived [other relatives], and many, many dear and devoted friends. [Name] was a [man/woman] of deep kindness, and [he/she] will be remembered for [his/her] constant smile. [Adjective], [nickname] [participated in hobby] into her final days, and we're sure that she is [participating in the hobby] in Heaven.

A celebration of life will be held at [time] on [date] at [location]. In lieu of flowers, please bring a little sunshine to our world, like [name] did, by making a donation to [charity].

[memorial quote]

Template 7: Medium contemporary

This is the same template as above, with optional details removed to fit a shorter format.

> [LAST NAME], [First name]. It is with a deep sense of sadness that the family of [name] announces [his/her] passing in [town] on [date]. [She/he] was predeceased in [year] by her [spouse/other important relatives].
>
> [Nickname] will be lovingly remembered by [children (spouses)]; and [grandchildren/great-grandchildren (spouses)].
>
> A celebration of life will be held at [time] on [date] at [location]. In lieu of flowers, please bring a little sunshine to our world, like [name] did, by making a donation to [charity].

Template 8: Religious Obituary

You can use this template on its own, or add lines from it to one of the other obituary templates.

> [LAST NAME], [First name]. On [date], [name] was called into the arms of the Lord and reunited with [important pre-deceased relatives]. [He/she] lived a rich live of dedicated service and [his/her] testimony will live on. A Memorial Service will be held on [date] at [location].
>
> "God saw you getting tired, and a cure was not to be.
> So He put His arms around you and whispered 'Come to ME'"

Template 9: Memorial (one or more years later)

A memorial usually consists of the person's name, their birth and death dates, a quote or verse, and a message of love. Instead of the verse, you can also just write your thoughts.

> [Name]. [Date of birth] – [Date of death]. We thought of you with love today, but that is nothing new; We thought of you yesterday: and days before that too. We thought of you in silence, we often speak your name: All we have is memories, and your picture in a frame. Your memory is our keepsake, with which we will never part: You are in good keeping; we have you in our hearts. We miss you and love you [name], and think of you every day. We will remember you always. Love, [family].

Made in the USA
Lexington, KY
24 July 2013